CONTENTS

INTRODUCTION

A comprehensive liquid diet surpasses the simplicity of tea or broth, offering highly nutritious alternatives. This specialized diet plays a vital role in both pre-procedural preparation and post-procedural healing, especially when solid food consumption is not feasible. Among the array of options available are savory soups, nourishing milk, comforting hot cereals, and revitalizing juices.

While the concept of a clear liquid diet, restricted to water, tea, and broth, might sound familiar, a full liquid diet expands on this notion. It encompasses all liquid-based foods or substances that naturally become liquid at room temperature or readily liquefy when exposed to body warmth. Consequently, this diet not only surpasses the nutritional value of a clear liquid diet but also promotes the body's recovery process following a medical procedure.

There are various circumstances under which your physician might recommend a full liquid diet, including:

- Preparation for a medical examination or procedure
- Post-surgical recovery, particularly after bariatric surgery
- Experiencing challenges with swallowing or chewing

Typically, individuals are advised to adhere to a full liquid diet for relatively short durations, such as five days to two weeks.

Now, let's delve deeper into the workings of this diet, explore the range of permissible foods, and highlight other crucial factors to consider.

A full liquid diet exclusively consists of fluids and foods that are naturally in liquid form or have the ability to transform into a liquid state at room temperature. This includes items like ice cream and milkshakes. Notably, a full liquid diet varies from a clear liquid diet, which restricts consumption to see-through foods like tea, broth, and gelatin.

The implementation of a full liquid diet can serve various purposes. It may be employed as a transitional phase after a gastrointestinal surgery or injury, following a clear liquid diet.

Additionally, it can be beneficial for individuals experiencing difficulties with swallowing or chewing.

This article delves into the advantages and potential drawbacks of a full liquid diet. It sheds light on the reasons why healthcare professionals may recommend it. Furthermore, a comprehensive list of foods to include and avoid is provided, along with valuable tips to ensure that your daily nutritional requirements are met.

Please note that all information provided is for general knowledge purposes only and should not substitute personalized medical advice.

CHAPTER ONE

It is important to note that liquid diets for weight loss purposes, especially highly restrictive ones, are not recommended by doctors as they can lead to nutritional deficiencies and weight regain once regular eating resumes.

A full liquid diet is an extension of the clear liquid diet, incorporating additional liquids like milk and small amounts of fiber. It is commonly used as a transitional phase between a clear liquid diet and a soft diet following gastrointestinal surgery or procedures. It can also be suitable for individuals with specific chewing and swallowing difficulties.

A properly planned full liquid diet provides adequate calories, protein, and fat. However, it may lack certain vitamins (such as vitamin B12, vitamin A, and thiamin), minerals (like iron), and fiber.

The following foods and liquids are typically allowed on a full liquid diet:

1. All foods permitted on the clear liquid diet: This includes popsicles, clear juice without pulp, plain gelatin, ice chips, water, sweetened tea or coffee (without creamer), clear broths, carbonated beverages, flavored water, and water.

2. Thin hot cereal or gruel: These can be consumed as long as they are adequately blended and strained.

3. Strained cream soups: Cream-based soups that have been strained to remove any solid particles are allowed.

4. Juices: Fruit juices, including nectars, are permitted on the full liquid diet.

5. Milkshakes: Milkshakes made with milk or dairy substitutes can be consumed.

6. Custard and puddings: These smooth and creamy desserts are suitable for a full liquid diet.

7. Liquid nutritional supplements: These products provide additional calories and nutrients and can be incorporated into the diet.

It is important to note that a full liquid diet should be well planned and may require supplementation to ensure proper intake of essential vitamins, minerals, and fiber. Consulting with a healthcare professional or registered dietitian is recommended to create an individualized full liquid diet plan.

What Is a Liquid Diet?

A liquid diet involves consuming most, if not all, of your calories from beverages rather than solid foods. There are different types of liquid diets, each serving a specific purpose.

1. Clear liquid diet: This type of diet is typically prescribed by a doctor for a short duration, usually before a medical procedure or to address certain digestive issues. It mainly consists of clear liquids such as water, broth, gelatin, and clear juices. However, it is low in calories and nutrients, so it should only be followed for a short period and under medical supervision.

2. Weight loss liquid diets: Some people opt for liquid diets as a way to lose weight. These diets often involve consuming fruit or vegetable juices, meal replacement shakes, or smoothies. In some cases, all meals are replaced with liquid options, while in others, only certain meals are substituted (commonly breakfast and lunch). Snacks may also be incorporated into the plan. These diets can help reduce calorie intake and promote weight loss, but they should not be followed for an extended period without medical guidance.

It's crucial to consult with a doctor before starting a liquid diet, regardless of the type. This ensures that you receive adequate essential nutrients like fiber and protein, which may be lacking in some liquid diets. Your doctor can guide you on how to maintain a balanced and healthy diet while meeting your specific nutritional needs.

Understanding the Mechanics of a Full Liquid Diet

The functionality of a full liquid diet revolves around the consumption of foods that are either already in liquid form or transform into a liquid state at room temperature. These liquid-based food choices are typically low in fiber and protein content, providing a respite for the digestive system.

To fulfill your caloric and nutrient requirements on a full liquid diet, you may need to consume more than the standard three meals per day. Aim for six to eight smaller meals throughout the day, incorporating a variety of liquids as well as strained or blended foods. To boost your calorie intake, consider adding full-fat dairy products like butter or whole milk, or opt for high-calorie supplement shakes.

For individuals concerned about obtaining complete nutrition on this diet, a liquid multivitamin can serve as a beneficial option.

Objectives of a Comprehensive Liquid Diet

The primary objective of a full liquid diet is to ensure sufficient nutrition intake while minimizing stress on the digestive system. However, this can be challenging due to certain digestive disorders that cause premature satiety or persistent nausea even after consuming small amounts of food.

To achieve the goals of a full liquid diet, it is crucial to focus on the following aspects:

1. Portion control: Consume enough food to feel satisfied while avoiding excessive strain on your system. Opt for several smaller meals throughout the day instead of three large ones.

2. Food selection: Include a variety of six or seven nutritionally dense foods in your diet. Consulting a registered dietitian or nutritionist can assist in making appropriate choices.

3. Nutritional tracking: Maintain a food diary to monitor your nutritional intake and utilize a nutrition app to calculate your daily calories, protein, and carbohydrate consumption.

Nutritional Targets

When properly balanced, a full liquid diet should provide approximately 1,500 calories and 45 grams of protein per day. This dietary approach is typically prescribed for only a few days to ease the transition back to a regular diet. Rarely does it extend beyond two weeks.

Exceptions may be made for individuals preparing for weight loss surgery, recovering from a fractured jaw, or managing chronic conditions like Crohn's disease.

Due to the restrictive nature of a full liquid diet, it is essential to have close supervision from a healthcare provider if adhering to this diet for more than a few days.

Reasons for Following a Full Liquid Diet

There are several reasons why you may be required to follow a full liquid diet. These include:

1. Medical Tests or Procedures: Prior to certain medical tests or procedures, such as colonoscopy or gastrointestinal imaging, a full liquid diet may be prescribed. Following the diet strictly is essential to ensure accurate test results and prevent complications during the procedure.

2. Pre-Surgery Preparation: Before specific types of surgery, including stomach or intestinal surgery, following a full liquid diet may be necessary. This helps to clear the digestive system, reduce the volume of the stomach and intestines, and minimize the risk of complications during surgery.

3. Post-Surgery Recovery: After undergoing stomach or intestinal surgery, a full liquid diet may be recommended during the initial stages of recovery. This allows the gastrointestinal system to heal gradually and reduces the strain on the

surgical site. The diet is gradually transitioned to more solid foods as tolerated.

4. Swallowing or Chewing Difficulties: Individuals who have trouble swallowing or chewing, known as dysphagia, may be prescribed a full liquid diet. This diet ensures that foods are in a form that can be easily consumed and digested without causing further discomfort or complications. Specific guidelines for the diet may be provided by a speech pathologist or healthcare professional.

5. Transition Diet: In some cases, a full liquid diet serves as an intermediate step between a clear liquid diet and a regular solid food diet. It allows for the gradual reintroduction of more substantial foods as the digestive system recovers or adjusts.

It is crucial to follow the prescribed full liquid diet accurately to achieve the intended goals, optimize recovery, and minimize the risks associated with specific medical procedures or conditions. It is recommended to consult with healthcare professionals or registered dietitians for personalized guidance and to address any concerns or questions.

Meal plan

A sample menu for a day on a full liquid diet could include:

Breakfast

- 1 cup of hot cereal (such as Cream of Wheat) diluted with whole milk

- 1/2 cup of fruit juice

Morning Snack

- 1/2 cup of a supplement beverage like Boost or Ensure
- 1/2 cup of custard-style yogurt

Lunch

- 2 cups of soup
- 1/2 cup of tomato juice
- 1 cup of chocolate pudding

Afternoon Snack

- 1/2 cup of a supplement beverage
- 1/2 cup of fruit juice

Dinner

- 2 cups of soup
- 1/2 to 1 cup of blended oatmeal diluted with milk
- 1/2 cup of lemonade

Evening Snack

- 1 cup of a supplement beverage
- 1/2 cup of vanilla ice cream

Sample meal 2

Breakfast:

- 1/2 cup of protein (e.g., pureed scrambled eggs or

> strained yogurt)

- 1/2 cup of skim milk
  - Option 1: Add 1/2 scoop of protein powder to the skim milk.
  - Option 2: Use 1/2 cup of meal replacement shake instead of skim milk.

Lunch:

- 1/2 cup of protein (e.g., pureed chicken or fish)
- 1/2 cup of fat-free yogurt (without added sugar)

Dinner:

- 1/2 cup of protein (e.g., pureed beef or tofu)
- 1/2 cup of strained, low-fat cream soup

Please note that this is just a sample menu, and individual dietary needs may vary. It is important to consult with a healthcare professional or registered dietitian to create a personalized full liquid diet plan that meets your specific requirements.

What Foods Can You eat

In comparison to a clear liquid diet, a full liquid diet offers a broader range of permissible food options. These include:

Fruits and Vegetables

- All fruit or vegetable juices (avoid pulp unless instructed otherwise by your doctor)

Soups

- Bouillon
- Clear broths (beef, chicken, vegetable)
- Strained and pureed vegetable soup
- Strained meat- or cream-based soups (may contain pureed vegetables or meat)

Dairy

- All types of cow's milk (whole, low-fat, reduced fat, fat-free)
- Lactose-free milk products such as soy, almond, or flax milk
- Half-and-half
- Butter
- Sour cream
- Custard-style yogurts

Grains

- Cream of Wheat
- Cream of Rice
- Grits
- Other cooked cereals made from refined grains and diluted with milk

Fats

- Butter

- Margarine
- Mayonnaise
- Creamy peanut butter or choice of nut butter

Beverages

- Coffee and tea
- Hot cocoa
- Artificially flavored fruit drinks
- Lemonade
- Sports drinks like Gatorade
- Milkshakes (you may add smooth peanut butter or canned fruit, but blend until smooth)
- Pasteurized eggnog

Supplement Beverages

- Ensure
- Boost
- Carnation Instant Breakfast
- Glucerna

Desserts

- Pudding
- Custard
- Gelatin
- Plain varieties of ice cream
- Sherbet

- Popsicles
- Fruit ices

Other

- Sweeteners such as honey, sugar, and maple syrup
- Salt
- Herbs, spices, and flavored syrups like chocolate syrup
- Brewer's yeast

Consult your doctor or dietitian regarding the following foods, as they may be included in a full liquid diet or become permissible as you approach a more regular diet:

- Pureed fruits like applesauce
- Pureed vegetables incorporated into soups, such as strained pumpkin puree in a cream soup
- Cooked cereals like oatmeal
- Pureed potatoes
- Strained, pureed meats

Foods to Avoid on a Full Liquid Diet

It is crucial to avoid solid foods entirely while adhering to a full liquid diet. This includes abstaining from raw, cooked, or canned fruits and vegetables that possess skins or seeds.

Other foods to steer clear of include:

- Mashed fruits and vegetables, like mashed avocado
- Nuts and seeds
- Hard and soft cheeses
- Soups containing noodles, rice, or other solid chunks
- Ice cream with solid additions
- Bread
- Whole cereals and grains
- Meats and meat substitutes
- Carbonated beverages such as sparkling water and soda

Individuals who have undergone stomach surgery may also need to avoid consuming orange and other acidic fruit and vegetable juices, as they can cause discomfort. If you have concerns about your vitamin C intake, consult your doctor regarding liquid vitamin C supplements.

Your doctor may provide additional dietary instructions based on the specific procedure you underwent.

Considerations before Starting a Full Liquid Diet

Your doctor serves as the primary resource for determining the foods suitable for your full liquid diet. Collaborating with a registered dietitian can also assist in planning your meals according to the guidelines of the diet while tailoring them to your specific needs. For instance, individuals with diabetes may require a specialized diet, and those who have undergone bariatric surgery may need to avoid or limit certain foods, such as sugar, on the full liquid diet for a specified duration.

Here are some additional factors to consider:

- Pureed foods should be of stage 1 consistency, resembling baby food without any visible pieces or chunks before blending them into soups and other liquids.

- Moistening foods with milk, water, salad dressings, or mayonnaise can facilitate the blending process.

- Pay attention to your body's signals of feeling full and stop drinking accordingly. Aim to consume at least 64 ounces of liquids per day.

- If you have difficulty drinking sufficient quantities, try consuming liquids in 15 to 20-minute intervals throughout the day.

- If you need to follow a full liquid diet for an extended period beyond five days, nutritional supplements may be recommended. Discuss the available options with your doctor.

- Consult your doctor or dietitian for specific menus and food ideas.

- It's important to note that following this type

of diet may result in rapid weight loss. It is intended for temporary use rather than long-term adoption, unless instructed otherwise by your doctor.

- Contact your doctor if you experience symptoms such as fever, diarrhea, vomiting, or abdominal pain while following a full liquid diet. These could indicate infection or other complications related to your surgery or medical condition.

Please note that all information provided is for general knowledge purposes only and should not substitute personalized medical advice.

General Advantages of a Comprehensive Liquid Diet

The full liquid diet offers several unique advantages, ensuring minimal strain on the gastrointestinal (digestive) system while providing enhanced flavor and nutritional value compared to a clear liquid diet.

This dietary approach eliminates the need for chewing and incorporates a range of fluids, including milk, fruit juices, shakes, and smoothies. It may also involve thicker options such as yogurt or puddings, ensuring they contain no lumps or solid components.

The primary objective of a full liquid diet is to facilitate the healing process of the entire digestive tract, encompassing the mouth, throat, colon, and rectum. Notably, this type of diet is not employed before gastrointestinal procedures like colonoscopy, which necessitate a clear liquid diet.

In contrast to a clear liquid diet, which only provides around 600 calories and 150 grams of carbohydrates per day, along with insufficient protein, vitamins, and minerals, the full liquid diet offers more substantial nutritional benefits. On average, adults in the United States require between 1,600 and 3,000 calories per day, as well as 225 to 325 grams of carbohydrates, to maintain normal bodily functions.

The full liquid diet encompasses nutritionally dense foods that are higher in protein and carbohydrates. While it may not fully meet your optimal nutritional needs, this diet serves as a temporary solution until you are capable of consuming soft or solid foods.

Indications for Implementing a Full Liquid Diet

Medical professionals may recommend a full liquid diet if you have specific medical conditions or are recovering from certain injuries or procedures.

The indications for a full liquid diet include:

1. Swallowing difficulties (dysphagia)
2. Chewing impairments
3. Severe mouth or throat ulcers
4. Jaw injuries
5. Digestive issues (such as gastroparesis and bowel strictures)
6. Recovery from gastrointestinal infections, injuries, or illnesses
7. Recovery from gastrointestinal, dental, oral, or weight loss surgeries

Side Effects of a Full Liquid Diet

Extended adherence to a full liquid diet can lead to certain side effects that should be taken into consideration. These effects include:

1. **Constipation**: Due to the limited intake of fiber, constipation may arise as a common issue. To alleviate symptoms, healthcare providers may recommend over-the-counter fiber supplements, such as Metamucil.
2. **Frequent Loose Stools**: The absence of solid foods in a full liquid diet can result in loose stools. However, as individuals transition back to a solid food diet, their bowel movements should normalize.
3. **Weight Loss**: Following a full liquid diet can lead to sudden and significant weight loss, even

in a short duration. To address this, healthcare providers may suggest high-calorie protein shakes, such as Ensure, to help regain weight once calorie intake increases.

4. **Nutritional Deficiencies**: As the diet provides fewer calories, vitamins, and minerals, individuals may experience symptoms of fatigue, irritability, depression, or general malaise. It is essential to communicate these symptoms to healthcare providers to explore potential solutions.

Risks of Full Liquid Diets

While a full liquid diet may be beneficial in specific situations, there are risks associated with long-term use or inadequate nutrition:

1. Nutritional Deficiencies: Full liquid diets may lack essential nutrients such as vitamin A, iron, vitamin B-12, and thiamine. Long-term adherence may require supplements to prevent deficiencies.

2. Limited Nutritional Variety: It can be challenging to obtain a diverse range of nutrients on a full liquid diet. Without proper planning and dietary knowledge, individuals may rely on less nutritious options, leading to inadequate nutrition.

3. Hunger and Mood Swings: The restrictive nature of a full liquid diet can lead to chronic hunger, mood swings, and reduced pleasure in eating.

4. Social Challenges: Participating in social activities centered around food or eating out can be difficult while on a full liquid diet, potentially impacting social interactions.

Recent research suggests that a full liquid diet may be more restrictive than necessary in some cases. Alternative options or less restrictive diets may be appropriate depending on the individual's condition and recovery progress.

When prescribed a full liquid diet, it is important to discuss concerns with the doctor and ask specific questions such as how to maintain health, the duration of the diet, associated risks, reasons for the recommendation, potential alternatives, and foods to avoid. Seeking guidance from a registered dietitian can also be beneficial.

Modifications to the Full Liquid Diet

Adjustments to the full liquid diet may be necessary based on age, overall health, and specific medical conditions. Some modifications include:

1. Post-Gastric Surgery: Acidic drinks like orange juice or coffee, which can irritate the stomach, may need to be avoided.

2. Kidney or Cardiovascular Disease: Fluid intake may require limitation to prevent fluid retention

and complications related to these conditions.

3. Diabetes: Extra precautions must be taken to manage blood sugar levels. Monitoring carbohydrate intake, which can raise blood sugar, is crucial.

4. Gastroparesis: Individuals with this condition, characterized by slow movement of food through the intestines, may need to avoid high-fat foods that are harder to digest.

5. Hypertension: Sodium (salt) intake may need to be limited for individuals with high blood pressure.

6. Lactose Intolerance: Those who are lactose intolerant should avoid cow's milk and other dairy products, seeking alternative sources of quality protein, calcium, and vitamin D.

Babies and Children

When implementing the full liquid diet for babies, toddlers, and children, additional adjustments may be required. For example, honey should not be given to children under one year of age. It is essential to consult with healthcare providers regarding appropriate milk consumption and consider adding electrolyte drinks or ice pops to prevent dehydration in cases of diarrhea.

Tips and Considerations

Following a full liquid diet may present challenges that require extra planning to incorporate liquid-only meals into daily life. Consider the following tips:

1. Practicality and Preparation: If you are recovering from an illness, injury, or surgery, you may not have the energy to prepare meals. Seek assistance from friends or family who are aware of your dietary restrictions. Preparing and freezing liquid meals in advance can also be beneficial. Consider purchasing necessary items, such as beverages and powder supplements, before starting the diet.

2. Cooking Tips: Thin soft foods by adding water or milk. Applying heat or using a microwave can help fully liquefy certain foods. Kitchen tools like food processors and blenders are useful for puréeing fruits, vegetables, and thickening foods like oatmeal.

3. Cost: While pre-puréed foods are available for purchase, they can be expensive and challenging to find. It may be more cost-effective to prepare puréed foods at home. Baby food can serve as a base for liquid meals, but may not provide sufficient portions for adults.

4. Nutritional Shakes: While nutritional shakes like Ensure and Glucerna may be costly, they can offer a substantial boost of protein and nutrition. However, they should not be relied upon as the sole source of nutrition.

Full Liquid Diet vs. Other Diets

A full liquid diet shares similarities with other diets used to treat digestive disorders or prepare for and recover from surgery. Here are some key differences:

1. Clear Liquid Diet: A clear liquid diet allows only fluids that are free of particles, typically employed before surgery or as part of colonoscopy preparation. It does not permit thick, opaque fluids.

2. Mechanical Soft Diets: A mechanical soft diet requires less chewing but may exclude certain soft foods based on texture or consistency. It is commonly recommended for healing from mouth, jaw, or throat injuries or surgeries, as well as post-illness recovery. A mechanical soft diet may be prescribed as a transition from a full liquid diet to regular solid foods.

3. Dysphagia Diet: Individuals with swallowing difficulties (dysphagia) may follow a three-stage diet, progressing from foods that don't require chewing to small, mashed or chopped solid pieces. The goal is to gradually reintroduce a regular solid food diet.

It is important to consult with healthcare professionals to determine the most suitable diet for specific conditions or recovery processes.

Uses of Full Liquid Diets

Doctors may recommend a full liquid diet in various situations, including:

1. Recovery from Pancreatitis: Following an episode of pancreatitis, a full liquid diet may be advised as the pancreas needs time to heal. This diet allows for easier digestion and reduces strain on the pancreas.

2. Transitional Diet after Weight Loss Surgery: After weight loss surgery, a full liquid diet is often recommended as an intermediate step between clear liquids and soft foods. It allows the stomach to heal and adjust to smaller food volumes.

3. Post-Dental or Oral Surgery: Individuals who have undergone dental or oral surgery may be advised to follow a full liquid diet for pain relief or when chewing solid foods is not possible. It ensures adequate nutrition while minimizing discomfort.

4. Post-Gastrointestinal Surgery or Digestive Disease Management: After gastrointestinal surgery or to manage symptoms of certain digestive diseases, a full liquid diet may be prescribed. It helps in providing necessary nutrients while allowing the digestive system to recover or cope with the condition.

5. Loss of Multiple Teeth or Jaw Injury: When multiple teeth are lost or there is a jaw injury, a full liquid diet can provide nutrition without the need for chewing solid foods.

6. Jaw Wired Shut: If the jaw is wired shut due to fractures or other medical reasons, a full liquid diet becomes essential to meet nutritional needs.

CHAPTER TWO

Fruit Smoothie made with Yogurt and Fresh Fruits

Description: Start your day with a refreshing and nutritious Fruit Smoothie made with creamy yogurt and a medley of fresh fruits. This vibrant smoothie is bursting with flavors and packed with vitamins and antioxidants.

Ingredients:

- 1 cup yogurt
- 1 banana
- 1 cup mixed berries (strawberries, blueberries, raspberries)
- 1/2 cup diced pineapple
- 1 tablespoon honey
- 1/2 cup ice cubes

Instructions:

1. In a blender, add yogurt, banana, mixed berries, diced pineapple, honey, and ice cubes.
2. Blend on high speed until smooth and creamy.
3. Pour into a glass and serve chilled.

Nutritional Information:

- Calories: 200
- Carbohydrates: 40g
- Protein: 8g
- Fat: 2g
- Fiber: 6g

Creamy Tomato Soup

Description: Indulge in the comforting goodness of Creamy Tomato Soup, a classic favorite. This velvety smooth soup is made with ripe tomatoes, aromatic herbs, and a touch of cream, resulting in a bowl of pure comfort.

Ingredients:

- 4 large tomatoes, diced
- 1 onion, chopped
- 2 garlic cloves, minced
- 2 tablespoons olive oil
- 1 cup vegetable broth
- 1/2 cup heavy cream
- Salt and pepper to taste

- Fresh basil leaves for garnish

Instructions:

1. Heat olive oil in a large pot over medium heat. Add chopped onions and minced garlic. Sauté until onions are translucent.

2. Add diced tomatoes and cook until they soften and release their juices.

3. Pour in vegetable broth and bring to a boil. Reduce heat and simmer for 15 minutes.

4. Using an immersion blender or a regular blender, puree the soup until smooth.

5. Return the soup to the pot and stir in the heavy cream. Season with salt and pepper to taste.

6. Cook for an additional 5 minutes, allowing the flavors to meld together.

7. Ladle the soup into bowls, garnish with fresh basil leaves, and serve hot.

Nutritional Information:

- Calories: 250
- Carbohydrates: 20g
- Protein: 5g
- Fat: 18g
- Fiber: 5g

Vanilla Protein Shake

Description: Kickstart your workout routine with a Vanilla

Protein Shake. This creamy and delicious shake is packed with protein, providing the fuel your body needs to recover and build lean muscle.

Ingredients:

- 1 scoop vanilla protein powder
- 1 cup unsweetened almond milk
- 1/2 frozen banana
- 1 tablespoon almond butter
- 1/2 teaspoon vanilla extract
- 1/2 cup ice cubes

Instructions:

1. In a blender, combine vanilla protein powder, unsweetened almond milk, frozen banana, almond butter, vanilla extract, and ice cubes.
2. Blend on high speed until smooth and creamy.
3. Pour into a glass and enjoy immediately.

Nutritional Information:

- Calories: 300
- Carbohydrates: 20g
- Protein: 30g
- Fat: 12g
- Fiber: 5g

Chicken Broth

Description: Chicken Broth is a comforting and nourishing soup that can be enjoyed on its own or used as a base for other recipes. Made with chicken bones, vegetables, and aromatic herbs, this homemade broth is rich in flavor and provides a soothing warmth.

Ingredients:

- 1 whole chicken, cut into pieces
- 2 carrots, chopped
- 2 celery stalks, chopped
- 1 onion, quartered
- 4 cloves of garlic, crushed
- Handful of fresh parsley
- 1 bay leaf
- Salt and pepper to taste
- Water

Instructions:

1. In a large pot, place the chicken pieces, carrots, celery, onion, garlic, parsley, and bay leaf.
2. Season with salt and pepper.
3. Pour enough water to cover all the ingredients in the pot.
4. Bring the mixture to a boil, then reduce the heat to low and let it simmer for 1-2 hours, skimming off any foam that rises to the top.

5. Remove the pot from heat and strain the broth, discarding the solids.

6. Let the broth cool down before storing in the refrigerator or using in recipes.

Nutritional Information:

- Calories: 120
- Carbohydrates: 2g
- Protein: 15g
- Fat: 6g
- Fiber: 0g

Vegetable Puree Soup

Description: Vegetable Puree Soup is a wholesome and flavorful dish that showcases the natural goodness of fresh vegetables. This smooth and velvety soup is a great way to increase your vegetable intake while enjoying a satisfying meal.

Ingredients:

- 2 carrots, peeled and chopped
- 2 zucchinis, chopped
- 1 leek, chopped
- 1 potato, peeled and diced
- 4 cups vegetable broth
- 1 tablespoon olive oil
- Salt and pepper to taste

- Fresh herbs for garnish (optional)

Instructions:

1. In a large pot, heat olive oil over medium heat. Add the chopped leek and sauté until softened.

2. Add the carrots, zucchinis, and potato to the pot. Stir and cook for a few minutes.

3. Pour in the vegetable broth and bring to a boil. Reduce the heat and simmer for 15-20 minutes, or until the vegetables are tender.

4. Using an immersion blender or regular blender, puree the soup until smooth.

5. Season with salt and pepper to taste.

6. Reheat the soup if needed and garnish with fresh herbs before serving.

Nutritional Information:

- Calories: 150

- Carbohydrates: 20g

- Protein: 3g

- Fat: 6g

- Fiber: 5g

Chocolate Banana Smoothie

Description: Indulge your sweet tooth with a Chocolate Banana Smoothie that tastes like a decadent treat but is actually good for you. This smoothie combines the richness of chocolate with the natural sweetness of bananas for a delightful and nutritious drink.

Ingredients:

- 1 ripe banana
- 1 cup almond milk
- 2 tablespoons cocoa powder
- 1 tablespoon honey or maple syrup
- 1/2 teaspoon vanilla extract
- 1/2 cup ice cubes

Instructions:

1. In a blender, combine the ripe banana, almond milk, cocoa powder, honey or maple syrup, vanilla extract, and ice cubes.
2. Blend on high speed until smooth and creamy.
3. Pour into a glass and enjoy immediately.

Nutritional Information:

- Calories: 180
- Carbohydrates: 35g
- Protein: 3g
- Fat: 5g
- Fiber: 5g

Cream of Mushroom Soup

Description: Indulge in the velvety richness of Cream of

Mushroom Soup, a comforting classic. This soup is made with earthy mushrooms, aromatic herbs, and a touch of cream to create a delightful blend of flavors and textures.

Ingredients:

- 8 ounces mushrooms, sliced
- 1 onion, chopped
- 2 cloves of garlic, minced
- 2 tablespoons butter
- 2 tablespoons all-purpose flour
- 4 cups vegetable broth
- 1 cup heavy cream
- Salt and pepper to taste
- Fresh parsley for garnish

Instructions:

1. In a large pot, melt the butter over medium heat. Add the chopped onion and minced garlic, sauté until fragrant.
2. Add the sliced mushrooms to the pot and cook until they release their moisture and become tender.
3. Sprinkle the flour over the mushrooms and stir well to coat.
4. Slowly pour in the vegetable broth while stirring continuously to avoid lumps.
5. Bring the mixture to a boil, then reduce the heat

and simmer for about 15 minutes.

6. Stir in the heavy cream and season with salt and pepper.

7. Continue to cook for an additional 5 minutes to heat through.

8. Ladle the soup into bowls, garnish with fresh parsley, and serve hot.

Nutritional Information:

- Calories: 250
- Carbohydrates: 12g
- Protein: 5g
- Fat: 20g
- Fiber: 2g

Mixed Berry Smoothie

Description: Treat yourself to a vibrant and refreshing Mixed Berry Smoothie packed with the goodness of antioxidant-rich berries. This colorful blend of fruits and yogurt provides a burst of flavors and a nourishing start to your day.

Ingredients:

- 1 cup mixed berries (strawberries, blueberries, raspberries)
- 1/2 cup plain yogurt
- 1/2 cup almond milk
- 1 tablespoon honey

- 1/2 teaspoon vanilla extract
- 1/2 cup ice cubes

Instructions:

1. In a blender, combine the mixed berries, plain yogurt, almond milk, honey, vanilla extract, and ice cubes.
2. Blend on high speed until smooth and creamy.
3. Pour into a glass and serve chilled.

Nutritional Information:

- Calories: 150
- Carbohydrates: 25g
- Protein: 6g
- Fat: 3g
- Fiber: 5g

Creamy Broccoli Soup

Description: Dive into a bowl of Creamy Broccoli Soup, a velvety blend of wholesome ingredients. This soup is packed with the goodness of nutrient-rich broccoli and creamy textures that will warm your soul.

Ingredients:

- 2 cups broccoli florets
- 1 onion, chopped
- 2 cloves of garlic, minced

- 2 tablespoons butter
- 3 cups vegetable broth
- 1 cup milk
- Salt and pepper to taste
- Grated cheddar cheese for garnish (optional)

Instructions:

1. In a large pot, melt the butter over medium heat. Add the chopped onion and minced garlic, sauté until fragrant.

2. Add the broccoli florets to the pot and cook for a few minutes until slightly softened.

3. Pour in the vegetable broth and bring to a boil. Reduce the heat and simmer for about 15 minutes or until the broccoli is tender.

4. Using an immersion blender or regular blender, puree the soup until smooth.

5. Return the soup to the pot and stir in the milk. Season with salt and pepper.

6. Heat the soup over low heat until warmed through.

7. Ladle the soup into bowls, garnish with grated cheddar cheese if desired, and serve hot.

Nutritional Information:

- Calories: 180
- Carbohydrates: 15g
- Protein: 6g

- Fat: 10g
- Fiber: 4g

Mango Lassi (Yogurt-Based Drink)

Description: Quench your thirst with the refreshing and tropical flavors of Mango Lassi. This yogurt-based drink combines the sweetness of ripe mangoes with a hint of tanginess for a delightful and creamy beverage.

Ingredients:

- 1 ripe mango, peeled and diced
- 1 cup plain yogurt
- 1/2 cup milk
- 1 tablespoon honey or sugar (optional)
- 1/4 teaspoon ground cardamom (optional)
- Ice cubes

Instructions:

1. In a blender, combine the diced mango, plain yogurt, milk, honey or sugar (optional), and ground cardamom (optional).
2. Blend on high speed until smooth and creamy.
3. Add ice cubes to the blender and blend again until the desired consistency is achieved.
4. Pour into glasses and serve chilled.

Nutritional Information:

- Calories: 180
- Carbohydrates: 30g
- Protein: 8g
- Fat: 4g
- Fiber: 3g

Butternut Squash Soup

Description: Cozy up with a bowl of Butternut Squash Soup, a velvety and nourishing dish that showcases the natural sweetness of this seasonal vegetable. The warm flavors and creamy texture make it a perfect comfort food.

Ingredients:

- 1 butternut squash, peeled, seeded, and cubed
- 1 onion, chopped
- 2 cloves of garlic, minced
- 2 tablespoons olive oil
- 4 cups vegetable broth
- 1/2 cup coconut milk
- 1/2 teaspoon ground cinnamon
- Salt and pepper to taste
- Roasted pumpkin seeds for garnish (optional)

Instructions:

1. Preheat the oven to 400°F (200°C).
2. Place the cubed butternut squash on a baking

sheet and drizzle with olive oil. Season with salt and pepper.

3. Roast the squash in the preheated oven for 30-40 minutes or until tender and caramelized.

4. In a large pot, heat olive oil over medium heat. Add the chopped onion and minced garlic, sauté until fragrant.

5. Add the roasted butternut squash to the pot and pour in the vegetable broth. Bring to a boil, then reduce the heat and simmer for 10-15 minutes.

6. Using an immersion blender or regular blender, puree the soup until smooth.

7. Stir in the coconut milk and ground cinnamon. Season with salt and pepper.

8. Heat the soup over low heat until warmed through.

9. Ladle the soup into bowls, garnish with roasted pumpkin seeds if desired, and serve hot.

Nutritional Information:

- Calories: 200
- Carbohydrates: 30g
- Protein: 5g
- Fat: 8g
- Fiber: 6g

Strawberry Yogurt Parfait

Description: Indulge in a delightful and nutritious Strawberry

Yogurt Parfait, a perfect combination of creamy yogurt, fresh strawberries, and crunchy granola. This parfait makes a satisfying breakfast or a healthy dessert option.

Ingredients:

- 1 cup plain Greek yogurt
- 1 cup fresh strawberries, sliced
- 1/2 cup granola
- 1 tablespoon honey or maple syrup (optional)

Instructions:

1. In a glass or jar, start layering the ingredients. Begin with a spoonful of Greek yogurt at the bottom.
2. Add a layer of sliced strawberries on top of the yogurt.
3. Sprinkle a layer of granola over the strawberries.
4. Repeat the layers until the glass or jar is filled.
5. Drizzle honey or maple syrup (optional) over the top layer.
6. Serve immediately and enjoy.

Nutritional Information:

- Calories: 250
- Carbohydrates: 30g
- Protein: 15g
- Fat: 8g

- Fiber: 5g

Creamy Spinach Soup

Description: Dive into a bowl of Creamy Spinach Soup, a velvety and vibrant dish packed with the goodness of nutrient-rich spinach. This soup is a perfect blend of flavors and textures, providing a comforting and nourishing meal.

Ingredients:

- 6 cups fresh spinach leaves
- 1 onion, chopped
- 2 cloves of garlic, minced
- 2 tablespoons butter
- 4 cups vegetable broth
- 1 cup milk or cream
- Salt and pepper to taste
- Nutmeg for garnish (optional)

Instructions:

1. In a large pot, melt the butter over medium heat. Add the chopped onion and minced garlic, sauté until fragrant.
2. Add the fresh spinach leaves to the pot and cook until wilted.
3. Pour in the vegetable broth and bring to a boil. Reduce the heat and simmer for about 10 minutes.

4. Using an immersion blender or regular blender, puree the soup until smooth.

5. Return the soup to the pot and stir in the milk or cream. Season with salt and pepper.

6. Heat the soup over low heat until warmed through.

7. Ladle the soup into bowls, garnish with a sprinkle of nutmeg if desired, and serve hot.

Nutritional Information:

- Calories: 180
- Carbohydrates: 12g
- Protein: 6g
- Fat: 12g
- Fiber: 4g

Avocado Smoothie

Description: Savor the creamy goodness of an Avocado Smoothie, a nutritious and filling drink that is both refreshing and satisfying. This smoothie combines the richness of ripe avocados with the tanginess of lime for a delightful flavor combination.

Ingredients:

- 1 ripe avocado, peeled and pitted
- 1 cup almond milk or any milk of your choice
- Juice of 1 lime

- 2 tablespoons honey or maple syrup
- 1/2 cup ice cubes

Instructions:

1. In a blender, combine the ripe avocado, almond milk or milk of your choice, lime juice, honey or maple syrup, and ice cubes.
2. Blend on high speed until smooth and creamy.
3. Pour into a glass and serve chilled.

Nutritional Information:

- Calories: 200
- Carbohydrates: 18g
- Protein: 3g
- Fat: 15g
- Fiber: 7g

Creamy Cauliflower Soup

Description: Indulge in a velvety bowl of Creamy Cauliflower Soup, a comforting and satisfying dish that highlights the delicate flavors of cauliflower. This soup is a perfect balance of creaminess and nourishment, making it a delightful choice for any occasion.

Ingredients:

- 1 head cauliflower, cut into florets
- 1 onion, chopped

- 2 cloves of garlic, minced
- 2 tablespoons butter or olive oil
- 4 cups vegetable broth
- 1 cup milk or cream
- Salt and pepper to taste
- Fresh chives for garnish (optional)

Instructions:

1. In a large pot, heat the butter or olive oil over medium heat. Add the chopped onion and minced garlic, sauté until fragrant.
2. Add the cauliflower florets to the pot and cook for a few minutes until slightly softened.
3. Pour in the vegetable broth and bring to a boil. Reduce the heat and simmer for about 15 minutes or until the cauliflower is tender.
4. Using an immersion blender or regular blender, puree the soup until smooth.
5. Return the soup to the pot and stir in the milk or cream. Season with salt and pepper.
6. Heat the soup over low heat until warmed through.
7. Ladle the soup into bowls, garnish with fresh chives if desired, and serve hot.

Nutritional Information:

- Calories: 180
- Carbohydrates: 14g

- Protein: 6g
- Fat: 10g
- Fiber: 6g

Coconut Milk-Based Curry Soup

Description: Experience the vibrant flavors of Coconut Milk-Based Curry Soup, a tantalizing blend of spices, vegetables, and creamy coconut milk. This soup brings together the richness of coconut with aromatic spices, creating a delightful and satisfying dish.

Ingredients:

- 1 tablespoon oil (such as olive oil or coconut oil)
- 1 onion, finely chopped
- 2 cloves of garlic, minced
- 1 tablespoon curry powder
- 1 teaspoon ground cumin
- 1 teaspoon ground coriander
- 1 teaspoon turmeric
- 1 can (13.5 oz) coconut milk
- 3 cups vegetable broth
- 1 cup diced vegetables of your choice (such as bell peppers, carrots, and zucchini)
- Salt and pepper to taste
- Fresh cilantro for garnish (optional)

Instructions:

1. Heat the oil in a large pot over medium heat. Add the chopped onion and minced garlic, sauté until fragrant.

2. Stir in the curry powder, cumin, coriander, and turmeric. Cook for 1-2 minutes to allow the spices to release their flavors.

3. Add the coconut milk and vegetable broth to the pot. Stir well to combine.

4. Bring the mixture to a simmer and let it cook for 10 minutes, allowing the flavors to meld together.

5. Add the diced vegetables to the pot and cook until they are tender but still slightly crisp.

6. Season with salt and pepper to taste.

7. Ladle the soup into bowls, garnish with fresh cilantro if desired, and serve hot.

Nutritional Information:

- Calories: 220
- Carbohydrates: 12g
- Protein: 3g
- Fat: 18g
- Fiber: 3g

Blueberry Kefir Smoothie

Description: Start your day on a vibrant note with a Blueberry Kefir Smoothie. This refreshing and probiotic-rich drink combines the tanginess of kefir with the sweetness of blueberries, creating a delightful and nutritious blend.

Ingredients:

- 1 cup blueberries (fresh or frozen)
- 1 cup kefir
- 1 tablespoon honey or maple syrup
- 1/2 teaspoon vanilla extract
- 1/2 cup ice cubes

Instructions:

1. In a blender, combine the blueberries, kefir, honey or maple syrup, vanilla extract, and ice cubes.
2. Blend on high speed until smooth and creamy.
3. Pour into a glass and serve chilled.

Nutritional Information:

- Calories: 150
- Carbohydrates: 20g
- Protein: 8g
- Fat: 4g
- Fiber: 3g

Creamy Asparagus Soup

Description: Indulge in the delicate flavors of Creamy Asparagus Soup, a velvety and nourishing dish that celebrates the essence of fresh asparagus. This soup is creamy, comforting, and perfect for showcasing the vibrant flavors of this seasonal vegetable.

Ingredients:

- 1 bunch asparagus, woody ends trimmed and chopped
- 1 onion, chopped
- 2 cloves of garlic, minced
- 2 tablespoons butter or olive oil
- 4 cups vegetable broth
- 1 cup milk or cream
- Salt and pepper to taste
- Lemon zest for garnish (optional)

Instructions:

1. In a large pot, melt the butter or heat the olive oil over medium heat. Add the chopped onion and minced garlic, sauté until fragrant.
2. Add the chopped asparagus to the pot and cook for a few minutes until slightly softened.
3. Pour in the vegetable broth and bring to a boil. Reduce the heat and simmer for about 15 minutes or until the asparagus is tender.
4. Using an immersion blender or regular blender, puree the soup until smooth.
5. Return the soup to the pot and stir in the milk or

cream. Season with salt and pepper.

6. Heat the soup over low heat until warmed through.

7. Ladle the soup into bowls, garnish with lemon zest if desired, and serve hot.

Nutritional Information:

- Calories: 160
- Carbohydrates: 12g
- Protein: 6g
- Fat: 10g
- Fiber: 4g

Watermelon Gazpacho

Description: Beat the heat with a refreshing Watermelon Gazpacho, a chilled soup bursting with the flavors of juicy watermelon and fresh vegetables. This light and tangy soup is perfect for hot summer days and provides a burst of hydration.

Ingredients:

- 4 cups diced watermelon
- 1 cucumber, peeled and diced
- 1 red bell pepper, seeded and diced
- 1 small red onion, chopped
- 2 tablespoons fresh lime juice
- 2 tablespoons extra-virgin olive oil

- 1 tablespoon fresh mint leaves, chopped
- Salt and pepper to taste

Instructions:

1. In a blender, combine the diced watermelon, cucumber, red bell pepper, red onion, lime juice, olive oil, and mint leaves.
2. Blend on high speed until smooth and well combined.
3. Season with salt and pepper to taste.
4. Transfer the gazpacho to a bowl and refrigerate for at least 1 hour to allow the flavors to meld together and the soup to chill.
5. Serve the gazpacho chilled in bowls or glasses. Garnish with additional mint leaves if desired.

Nutritional Information:

- Calories: 80
- Carbohydrates: 10g
- Protein: 1g
- Fat: 4g
- Fiber: 2g

Green Detox Smoothie

Description: Revitalize your body with a Green Detox Smoothie, a vibrant blend of nutrient-packed greens and refreshing fruits. This smoothie is loaded with vitamins and antioxidants, making it a perfect choice for a healthy and energizing start to your day.

Ingredients:

- 1 cup spinach leaves
- 1 cup kale leaves
- 1/2 cucumber, peeled and sliced
- 1 green apple, cored and chopped
- 1/2 ripe banana
- 1 cup coconut water or water
- Juice of 1/2 lemon
- 1 tablespoon chia seeds (optional)
- Ice cubes

Instructions:

1. In a blender, combine the spinach leaves, kale leaves, cucumber, green apple, ripe banana, coconut water or water, lemon juice, and chia seeds (optional).
2. Blend on high speed until smooth and creamy.
3. Add ice cubes to the blender and blend again until the desired consistency is achieved.
4. Pour into a glass and serve chilled.

Nutritional Information:

- Calories: 120
- Carbohydrates: 28g

- Protein: 4g
- Fat: 2g
- Fiber: 8g

Creamy Carrot Soup

Description: Warm up with a bowl of Creamy Carrot Soup, a velvety and nourishing dish that highlights the natural sweetness of carrots. This soup is smooth, comforting, and packed with vitamins, making it a perfect choice for a satisfying meal.

Ingredients:

- 4 cups sliced carrots
- 1 onion, chopped
- 2 cloves of garlic, minced
- 2 tablespoons butter or olive oil
- 4 cups vegetable broth
- 1 cup milk or cream
- Salt and pepper to taste
- Fresh parsley for garnish (optional)

Instructions:

1. In a large pot, melt the butter or heat the olive oil over medium heat. Add the chopped onion and minced garlic, sauté until fragrant.
2. Add the sliced carrots to the pot and cook for a few

minutes until slightly softened.

3. Pour in the vegetable broth and bring to a boil. Reduce the heat and simmer for about 15 minutes or until the carrots are tender.

4. Using an immersion blender or regular blender, puree the soup until smooth.

5. Return the soup to the pot and stir in the milk or cream. Season with salt and pepper.

6. Heat the soup over low heat until warmed through.

7. Ladle the soup into bowls, garnish with fresh parsley if desired, and serve hot.

Nutritional Information:

- Calories: 160
- Carbohydrates: 14g
- Protein: 4g
- Fat: 10g
- Fiber: 4g

Kiwi and Spinach Smoothie

Description: Energize your day with a Kiwi and Spinach Smoothie, a vibrant and nutrient-packed blend of fresh kiwi, spinach, and other wholesome ingredients. This smoothie is a refreshing way to incorporate greens into your diet while enjoying a delightful burst of tropical flavors.

Ingredients:

- 2 ripe kiwis, peeled and chopped
- 1 cup fresh spinach leaves
- 1 ripe banana
- 1/2 cup Greek yogurt
- 1 tablespoon honey or maple syrup
- 1/2 cup almond milk or any milk of your choice
- Ice cubes

Instructions:

1. In a blender, combine the chopped kiwis, spinach leaves, ripe banana, Greek yogurt, honey or maple syrup, and almond milk.
2. Blend on high speed until smooth and creamy.
3. Add ice cubes to the blender and blend again until the desired consistency is achieved.
4. Pour into a glass and serve chilled.

Nutritional Information:

- Calories: 180
- Carbohydrates: 38g
- Protein: 7g
- Fat: 2g
- Fiber: 6g

Creamy Potato Soup

Description: Indulge in a bowl of comforting Creamy Potato Soup, a hearty and satisfying dish that highlights the creamy goodness of potatoes. This soup is rich, velvety, and packed with flavors that will warm you from the inside out.

Ingredients:

- 4 large potatoes, peeled and diced
- 1 onion, chopped
- 2 cloves of garlic, minced
- 2 tablespoons butter or olive oil
- 4 cups vegetable broth
- 1 cup milk or cream
- Salt and pepper to taste
- Fresh chives for garnish (optional)

Instructions:

1. In a large pot, melt the butter or heat the olive oil over medium heat. Add the chopped onion and minced garlic, sauté until fragrant.

2. Add the diced potatoes to the pot and cook for a few minutes until slightly softened.

3. Pour in the vegetable broth and bring to a boil. Reduce the heat and simmer for about 20 minutes or until the potatoes are tender.

4. Using an immersion blender or regular blender, puree half of the soup to create a creamy base while still leaving some chunks of potatoes for

texture.

5. Return the soup to the pot and stir in the milk or cream. Season with salt and pepper.

6. Heat the soup over low heat until warmed through.

7. Ladle the soup into bowls, garnish with fresh chives if desired, and serve hot.

Nutritional Information:

- Calories: 220

- Carbohydrates: 38g

- Protein: 6g

- Fat: 6g

- Fiber: 4g

Pea and Mint Soup

Description: Delight in the fresh flavors of Pea and Mint Soup, a vibrant and invigorating dish that combines the sweetness of peas with the refreshing aroma of mint. This soup is light, nutritious, and perfect for celebrating the flavors of spring.

Ingredients:

- 2 cups fresh or frozen peas

- 1 onion, chopped

- 2 cloves of garlic, minced

- 2 tablespoons butter or olive oil

- 4 cups vegetable broth
- 1/2 cup fresh mint leaves, chopped
- Salt and pepper to taste
- Greek yogurt for garnish (optional)

Instructions:

1. In a large pot, melt the butter or heat the olive oil over medium heat. Add the chopped onion and minced garlic, sauté until fragrant.

2. Add the peas to the pot and cook for a few minutes until heated through.

3. Pour in the vegetable broth and bring to a boil. Reduce the heat and simmer for about 10 minutes.

4. Stir in the chopped mint leaves.

5. Using an immersion blender or regular blender, puree the soup until smooth.

6. Season with salt and pepper to taste.

7. Heat the soup over low heat until warmed through.

8. Ladle the soup into bowls, swirl in some Greek yogurt if desired, and serve hot.

Nutritional Information:

- Calories: 180
- Carbohydrates: 26g
- Protein: 7g
- Fat: 6g

- Fiber: 8g

Chilled Cucumber and Yogurt Soup

Description: Beat the summer heat with a refreshing Chilled Cucumber and Yogurt Soup. This cooling soup combines the crispness of cucumbers with the creamy tanginess of yogurt, creating a light and satisfying dish that will leave you feeling refreshed.

Ingredients:

- 2 large cucumbers, peeled and chopped
- 1 cup Greek yogurt
- 1/4 cup fresh mint leaves, chopped
- 2 tablespoons lemon juice
- 1 clove of garlic, minced
- 1 tablespoon extra-virgin olive oil
- Salt and pepper to taste
- Cucumber slices and mint leaves for garnish (optional)

Instructions:

1. In a blender, combine the chopped cucumbers, Greek yogurt, fresh mint leaves, lemon juice, minced garlic, and extra-virgin olive oil.
2. Blend on high speed until smooth and well combined.
3. Season with salt and pepper to taste.

4. Transfer the soup to a bowl and refrigerate for at least 1 hour to allow the flavors to meld together and the soup to chill.

5. Serve the chilled cucumber and yogurt soup in bowls or glasses. Garnish with cucumber slices and mint leaves if desired.

Nutritional Information:

- Calories: 100
- Carbohydrates: 10g
- Protein: 7g
- Fat: 5g
- Fiber: 2g

CONCLUSION

Adhering to a full liquid diet can indeed pose challenges. If an individual needs to follow this diet for an extended period, it is advisable to consult a dietitian to ensure proper intake of essential nutrients.

In many instances, it is feasible to maintain a satisfying and nutritious diet by pureeing the foods one typically enjoys. Pureeing allows for the consumption of familiar flavors and textures while still adhering to the requirements of a full liquid diet.

Working with a dietitian can provide valuable guidance on creating a well-rounded pureed diet that meets individual nutritional needs. They can offer suggestions on food choices, recipes, and techniques to ensure a balanced intake of important nutrients.

By pureeing a variety of foods, individuals can diversify their diet and minimize monotony. This approach can help enhance compliance with the full liquid diet while maintaining enjoyment and satisfaction with meals.

Remember, consulting a dietitian is key to developing a personalized and nutritionally sound pureed diet plan.